Kidney Stone Buster:
The Quick Guide to Prevent Stones Fast

BY

DR ANTHONY DAT

Copyright © 2025 Anthony Dat

All rights reserved.

No part of this book may be reproduced, distributed, or transmitted in any form without permission, except for brief quotations used in reviews or academic references.

Medical disclaimer

This book provides general health information for educational purposes only and is not a substitute for individual medical advice. Always consult a qualified healthcare professional before making changes to your diet, medications, supplements, or lifestyle. The author accepts no liability for outcomes arising from the use of this book.

For Flora and Penny,

who make everything worthwhile,

with love and gratitude always.

Table of Contents

A note to readers 7

Introduction 9

Chapter 1: Understanding Kidney Stones 13

Chapter 2: Hydration 19

Chapter 3: Diet 23

Chapter 4: Safe Foods and Food Swaps 29

Chapter 5: Simple Kidney-Friendly Recipes 33

Chapter 6: Lifestyle Modification 41

Chapter 7: The 4 Week Stone Free Plan 47

Chapter 8: Staying Stonefree for Life 51

About the Author 55

A note to readers

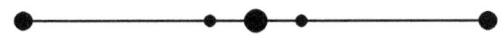

This book is designed to support and educate you about kidney stone prevention, drawing on current medical knowledge and the author's clinical experience. It is not intended to replace your own personal medical care.

Everyone's health situation is different. Before making changes to your diet, fluid intake, medications, or supplements, it is important to discuss these with your general practitioner, local doctor, urologist or another qualified health professional who knows your individual circumstances. The author cannot take responsibility for outcomes related to how the information is applied.

If you experience severe pain, fever, vomiting, or blood in the urine, please seek urgent medical attention.

Thank you for taking an active role in your kidney health.

Introduction

If you have ever experienced a kidney stone attack then you know how horrible the pain can be. The intense, excruciating pain is something like no other. Kidney stone pain is unfortunately relatively common, with an estimated 1 in 10 people suffering from kidney stones at some point in their life. The good news, however, is that for the most part, **kidney stones are largely preventable**.

With the right knowledge of diet, fluid intake, and lifestyle changes, you can lower your risk of developing them. In this book, I will share simple tips and tricks with you from my years working as a Urological Surgeon to help you prevent kidney stones from forming naturally.

Kidney Stones: The 'gift' that keeps on giving

Kidney stones are not only annoying, but they can also come back repeatedly. In fact, up to 50% of kidney stone sufferers will have another episode within 5 to 10 years. This cycle of pain is costly and frustrating on multiple levels – physically, emotionally, and financially. You may have heard conflicting advice about what prevention options work. The question, though, is what actually works and is backed by science?

The Truth About Prevention

Preventing kidney stones does not have to be complicated. The key to prevention lies in three simple prevention pillars:

1. **Hydration**
2. **Diet and Nutrition**
3. **Lifestyle Habits**

Throughout this book, I will show you each of these pillars, providing you with **easy to follow strategies** that will reduce your risk of developing a kidney stone. You will learn about which foods and fluids to embrace and the habits to build and change in your regular daily routine.

Who This Book Is For

This book is for anyone who wants to prevent kidney stones. Whether you have already experienced the agony of passing a kidney stone or you simply want to learn how to support your kidneys for better overall health, this book will equip you with the knowledge to succeed.

How This Book Is Structured

This isn't just another health book with vague tips and theories. What you'll find here are **practical, science-based strategies** that have been shown to help people prevent kidney stones. We will explore:

- The role of water and hydration in kidney stone prevention
- How diet impacts your stone forming risk

- The lifestyle factors, such as sleep and stress management, that make a significant difference

To make the process as easy as possible, I have designed a **4 week plan** that introduces each of these pillars in a gradual approach that you can build into a sustainable, kidney stone-free lifestyle long-term.

Are you ready to take charge of your kidney health? Let's get started!

Chapter 1:
Understanding Kidney Stones

Kidney stones are one of the most common kidney conditions. In this chapter, we will explore what kidney stones are, including the different types, risk factors, and symptoms.

What Are Kidney Stones?

Kidney stones, also known as renal stones or nephrolithiasis, are solid crystal stones that form inside the kidneys from substances found in urine. Urine contains a variety of waste products, such as acids, salts, and minerals, which are filtered by the kidneys. When the balance of these products is disrupted, some can begin to crystallise and form stones.

The stone size may vary from a few millimetres to a full cast of the kidney collecting system (known as a staghorn calculus). The stones start causing pain when they start moving down the urine tube (ureter) causing a blockage.

Types of Kidney Stones

There are four main types of kidney stones made of different substances. Understanding the type of stone can help you prevent future occurrences of stones:

1. **Calcium Oxalate Stones**
   - o **Most common** stone type, making up to **80%** of kidney stones. They form when calcium combines with oxalate (a naturally occurring substance in certain foods) to create crystals.
   - o **Cause**: These stones often form due to high calcium levels in the urine, low urine volume, or high intake from oxalate-rich foods such as spinach and certain nuts.

2. **Uric Acid Stones**
   - o **Caused by excess uric acid**: These stones develop when there is too much uric acid in the urine, often due to a high-protein diet or gout.
   - o **Risk Factors**: Obesity, dehydration, and certain metabolic disorders can increase uric acid levels.

3. **Struvite Stones**
   - o **Infection-related**: These are often caused by chronic urinary tract infections (UTIs), where bacteria produce ammonia that mixes with magnesium and phosphate to form struvite crystals.

4. **Cystine Stones**
   - o **Genetic condition**: Cystine stones are rare. It forms in people with a genetic disorder called cystinuria, which causes excess cystine (an amino acid protein) to be excreted in the urine.

- o **Challenges**: This condition has a high tendency to occur and usually requires a multidisciplinary team approach with a nephrologist (kidney physician) and dietician to manage.

How Kidney Stones Form

Kidney stones occur when there is an excess of some substances in urine, such as calcium, uric acid, oxalate, and phosphate. These will begin to accumulate and cause crystal formation.

Risk Factors for Kidney Stones

Kidney stones can be predisposed to several things. Such as:

- **Diet**: Consumption and intake of large quantities of animal protein, sugar, and salt and insufficient amounts of fibre can lead to kidney stones. High-oxalate foods like spinach and beets also contribute to the formation of the stones.
- **Dehydration**: Lack of water causes the urine to be more concentrated, which increases the risk of kidney stones.
- **Obesity**: Overweight or obese individuals usually contain more calcium, uric acid and oxalate in their urine.
- **Family History**: You have a higher chance of getting kidney stones should you have a family history of kidney stones.
- **Other Medical Conditions**: Diseases causing increased excretion of uric acid, calcium, and oxalate can increase your risk of getting stones. These include hyperparathyroidism, gout, and Crohn's disease.
- **Medications and Supplements**: Certain drugs, such as diuretics, increase the risk of getting kidney stones.

Symptoms of Kidney Stones

The most common symptom of a kidney stone is sharp, intense pain that comes and goes ('colicky'). This pain often starts in the flank region and radiates towards to groin. Other symptoms include:

- **Nausea and vomiting**: Kidney stone pain can be so intense that it may trigger nausea or vomiting.

- **Blood in the urine**: You may notice pink, red, or brown urine due to stone passage.

- **Frequent urination**: You may feel the urge to urinate frequently, especially if the stone is near the bladder.

- **Cloudy or foul-smelling urine with fevers and chills**: This can be a sign of a concurrent infection. If you feel feverish with a suspected kidney stone, you must present to your closest emergency department. This is because an **obstructing kidney stone with an infection** is a urological emergency and needs to be drained as soon as possible.

Why Kidney Stones Keep Coming Back

The risk of developing more kidney stones is higher once you have had one stone. As highlighted previously, **50%** of people who've had a stone will experience another episode within **5 to 10 years**. The question is - why do so many come back with stones?

There are several reasons:

- **Diet, fluid, and lifestyle habits**: Many people continue with the same eating habits and low fluid intake that led to their first stone, which increases their risk for recurrence.

- **Underlying conditions**: Certain medical conditions, such as gout and hyperparathyroidism, can make you more susceptible to stones.
- **Genetics**: Genetically, some individuals are more prone to form stones, meaning they may need more careful management of fluid, diet, and lifestyle factors.

Conclusion

Kidney stones are painful and often recurrent. With the right approach, however, **you can prevent them**. Because kidney stones vary in composition, prevention strategies can differ depending on stone type, medical conditions, and individual risk factors. In Chapter 2, we will explore one of the most important strategies for effectively preventing kidney stones: **maximising hydration**.

Chapter 2:
Hydration

The biggest takeaway from this book is that **adequate hydration is the single most effective natural way to prevent kidney stones.** Adequate hydration flushes out waste products and dilutes stone-forming minerals.

Why Dehydration Leads to Stones

Your kidneys are designed to filter waste products from your blood and expel them in your urine. But if there isn't enough fluid available, the urine becomes concentrated—like a muddy river instead of a flowing stream. In this dense environment, minerals such as calcium and oxalate can clump together and crystallise. That is the initial step in the formation of kidney stones.

How Much Water Do You Actually Need?

At least **2.5 to 3 litres (10-12 cups) of fluids daily.** More if you sweat heavily, exercise, or live in a hot climate.

Despite this, you can still 'over-do' hydration. Drinking excessive amounts of water (greater than 1 litre per hour for a number of hours) in a short period can be dangerous. This may lead to low blood sodium levels (hyponatraemia), which is a serious medical condition. Aim for regular, steady hydration throughout the day rather than large volumes all at once.

People with fluid overload conditions such as congestive heart failure, liver cirrhosis, or chronic kidney disease should follow individualised fluid advice from their treating doctor, as fluid requirements and restrictions may differ.

Tip: The best way to know if you are well hydrated is by looking at your urine. It should look pale yellow or clearer, with no smell. Another good sign is not feeling thirsty.

Best Fluids for Kidney Stone Prevention

The best fluid is plain water.

Great Choices:

- **Water (still or sparkling)** – The best
- **Citrus juices** – Citrate is abundant in citrus juices (such as lemon or lime juice) and prevents the formation of stones.

Good in Moderation:

- **Coffee and tea**
- **Milk or calcium-fortified plant milks**

Avoid or Limit:

- **Carbonated soft drinks** – Contain phosphoric acid, which may promote stones
- **Excess alcohol** – Dehydrates and disrupts kidney function

The Citrate Connection

Citrate is a natural compound found in citrus fruits. It plays a protective role by binding with calcium in urine, preventing it from combining with oxalate or phosphate. Increasing natural levels of citrate may be achieved by adding lemon or lime juice to your water.

Try:

- Adding **2 tablespoons of lemon juice** to a glass of water, 2–3 times a day
- Drinking **diluted lemonade** (low-sugar) throughout the day

How to Make Hydration a Habit

The habit of drinking more water during the day can be hard. These are effective strategies that can make you stay hydrated all the time:

1. Start Your Day with Water

Take a glass of water as the first thing in the morning before coffee or any other drink.

2. Use a Measured Bottle

Purchase a 1- or 2-litre (s) water bottle as a guide to keep track of fluid intake per day.

3. Set Reminders

An hourly reminder can be set by phone to ensure regular fluid intake.

4. Flavour It Naturally

You can add cucumber, lemon, berries or mint to your water to add variety.

5. Drink Before You're Thirsty

The thirst comes late – aim to continuously sip over the course of the day.

Takeaway Tips

- Aim for **2.5 to 3 litres of fluid per day** to produce 2+ litres of urine
- Water is best
- Avoid sugary sodas and excess caffeine
- Make hydration automatic with bottles, reminders, and building good habits
- Drinking too much water is also not good and patients with fluid overload conditions should seek individualised advice from their doctor.
- Listen to your body. You are well hydrated if you are not feeling thirsty and your urine is pale yellow or clearer with no smell.

Chapter 3:
Diet

Your diet has a large influence on kidney stone formation and recurrence. In this chapter, we will explore the many different ways you can reduce your stone risk.

The Big Picture: Balance Over Restriction

The key is to ensure diet moderation with the following goals:

- **Moderate** high-risk stone forming foods
- **Pair** certain foods to reduce absorption of stone-forming compounds
- **Add** more protective foods to your plate

Step 1: Don't Fear Calcium—Include It Wisely

It sounds counterintuitive, but **low calcium intake can increase your risk** of kidney stones—especially calcium oxalate stones. Why? Dietary calcium **binds with oxalate in your gut**, preventing it from being absorbed and excreted through the kidneys.

Smart Calcium Guidelines:

- Aim for **1,000–1,200 mg per day** from food (not supplements unless prescribed)
- Include calcium **with meals**, especially those that contain oxalate

Best sources:

- Low-fat milk or yoghurt
- Calcium-fortified plant milks
- Tofu set with calcium
- Canned salmon or sardines (with bones)

Step 2: Control Oxalate, Don't Eliminate It

Oxalate is a natural substance found in many healthy foods. Despite this, too much oxalate can predispose to calcium oxalate stones.

High oxalate foods:

- Spinach
- Beets
- Almonds
- Rhubarb

- Swiss chard
- Dark chocolate
- Sweet potatoes

Pro tip: Eat these with calcium-rich foods. For example, a small spinach salad with a serving of low-fat cheese helps calcium bind to oxalate in your gut—so less ends up in your urine.

Step 3: Reduce Salt

Salt increases calcium excretion in the urine. The more sodium you consume, the more calcium your kidneys flush out—and that extra calcium can combine with oxalate or phosphate to form stones.

Simple ways to reduce sodium:

- Cook from scratch
- Limit processed foods, deli meats, and canned soups
- Choose "low sodium" or "no added salt" versions of packaged foods
- Use herbs, lemon, and spices instead of the salt shaker

Goal: Stay under **2,300 mg of sodium per day**, or ideally **1,500 mg per day** if you've had stones before.

Step 4: Eat the Right Amount of Protein

Animal protein—like red meat, poultry, fish, and eggs—can increase **uric acid** and lower **citrate**, all of which increase stone risk.

You don't have to go vegetarian, but you should:

- Limit animal protein to **1–2 servings per day**

- Add plant proteins such as beans, lentils, tofu, and quinoa
- Select lean cuts and smaller portions

Step 5: Cut Back on Sugar—Especially Fructose

Fructose contained in sodas and sweets increases the risk of kidney stones. It promotes higher amounts of calcium, oxalate and uric acid concentration in the urine.

High sugar beverages/foods:

- Soft drinks, especially cola
- Lollies, sweet baked goods, and energy bars
- Fruit juice and sweetened yoghurts

Better choices: Whole fruits, plain yoghurt with berries, and unsweetened beverages.

Step 6: Load Up on Fruits and Veggies

Potassium, magnesium, and citrate, which are found in vegetables and fruits, are useful in the prevention of the formation of kidney stones. Citrate especially attaches calcium in urine, preventing it from forming crystals.

Focus on:

- Lemons, limes, oranges
- Bananas, melons, and avocados
- Potatoes (with skin), squash, and peppers
- Leafy greens (not spinach)

Have no less than 5 servings of vegetables and fruits per day. They are also useful in reducing the acidity of your urine, which is significant in the prevention of uric acid and cystine stones.

Step 7: Mind Your Oxalate–Calcium Timing

One of the most neglected but most effective methods to prevent kidney stones is the combination of foods. By eating a combination of high-oxalate and foods high in calcium, the calcium neutralises the oxalate in the intestines. This prevents the oxalate from entering the kidneys.

Examples:

- Add a low-fat milk to oatmeal and almond butter.
- Adding low fat cheese with spinach
- Serve sweet potato with fresh yoghurt

What About Supplements?

Some supplements increase risk, such as:

- **Vitamin C (ascorbic acid)**: With large dosage (above 1000 mg/day), it can be oxidised to oxalate.
- **Vitamin D:** Generally safe at moderate doses, but high doses — especially when combined with calcium supplements — may increase stone risk. People with kidney stones should discuss vitamin D use with their doctor.
- **Calcium supplements**: Too much calcium can increase the amount of calcium excretion in the urine causing stones.
- **Protein powders**: These are rich in oxalate or acid-forming compounds.

Tip: Never take up supplements unless you have spoken with a doctor, especially when you have had a previous history of stones.

The Oxalate Myth: You Don't Need to Go to Extremes

A large number of individuals attempt low-oxalate diets and end up unnecessarily cutting out healthy foods. Don't to this! Instead, you should:

- Pair high oxalate foods with calcium foods
- Drink enough water
- Reduce salt and animal protein intake

That combination is more effective—and more realistic—than banning oxalate foods long-term.

Takeaway Tips

- **Eat 3 servings of calcium-rich foods daily**, with meals
- **Pair calcium with oxalate** when eating high-oxalate foods
- **Limit sodium** to under 2,300 mg/day
- **Go easy on animal protein**—swap in plant proteins
- **Cut sugary drinks** and processed foods
- **Eat a rainbow** of fruits and vegetables daily
- Avoid extreme diets—**balance is best**

Chapter 4:
Safe Foods and Food Swaps

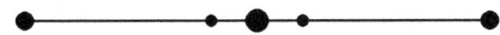

This chapter will focus on easy food replacements for high-risk stone forming foods to enhance your everyday habits.

What Does "Kidney-Safe" Mean?

'Kidney Safe' foods are those that are:

- Low in oxalate (or easy to pair with calcium)
- Low in added sugar and sodium
- Not acid-forming (or buffered with fruits/vegetables)
- Supportive of citrate levels, fluid intake, or urine pH

We are going to look at those foods that can be considered in these rules and how you can make a plan for a week around these foods.

Top 12 Stone-Safe Foods to Eat Freely

1. **Cucumbers**
2. **Capsicum**
3. **Cauliflower**
4. **Bananas** – They contain much potassium and very little oxalate. They serve as excellent snacks either eaten alone or put in yummy smoothies!
5. **Melons (cantaloupe, watermelon, honeydew)**
6. **Brown rice** – Less oxalate content compared to white rice, and regulates blood glucose.
7. **Tofu (calcium-set)**
8. **Lentils** – Vegetable protein with high levels of fibre, magnesium, and potassium.
9. **Low-fat plain yogurt** – It provides calcium and good gut probiotics.
10. **Oats** – Low oxalate and high fibre are good breakfast foods.
11. **Citrus fruits (lemons, limes, oranges)**
12. **Herbs and spices (ginger, basil, turmeric)**

Smart Swaps to Make Your Diet Stone-Safe

Instead of...	Try this...	Why it helps
Spinach salad	Romaine or arugula	Leafy greens that have lower levels of oxalate
Almonds	Walnuts or macadamias	Lower oxalate, healthy nuts
Cola	Carbonated water with squeeze of lemon	Stay away from phosphoric acid
White bread	Wholegrain	High in fibre and better blood glucose control
Red meat	Grilled tofu or lentils	Less acidic
Soy sauce	Low-sodium tamari	Reduced sodium
Potato chips	Air-popped popcorn	Lower oxalate, less sodium
Processed deli meat	Grilled chicken or turkey slices	Less salt, fewer additives
Fruit juice	Whole fruit + water	Fibre plus slower sugar release

Simple Sample Meal Ideas

Breakfast:

- Oatmeal with banana and cinnamon
- Whole-grain toast with avocado
- Yoghurt with fresh berries and flaxseed

Lunch:

- Quinoa salad with cucumber, capsicum, and lemon vinaigrette
- Lentil soup with a whole grain roll

- Turkey and spinach-free veggie wrap with hummus

Dinner:

- Roasted cauliflower, brown rice and grilled salmon.
- Tofu stir-fry in broccoli and carrots and light soy sauce.
- Baked Sweet potato mixed with low-fat cottage cheese and herbs.

Snacks:

- Fresh melon slices
- Handful of walnuts
- Carrot sticks with tahini dip
- Unsweetened herbal tea and whole grain crackers

Takeaway Tips

- Focus on real, whole foods low in oxalate and sodium
- Make swaps, not sacrifices—small changes add up
- Eat high-oxalate foods with foods that contain calcium
- Attempt to eat a balanced plate containing plant protein, good fats and fibre.

Chapter 5:
Simple Kidney-Friendly Recipes

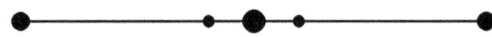

The following kidney friendly recipes are easy to prepare, family friendly and budget conscious:

Breakfasts

1. Lemon and Blueberry Overnight Oats

Ingredients:

- ½ cup rolled oats
- ½ cup coconut milk or low fat cow's milk
- ¼ cup yoghurt
- 1 tbsp ground chia seeds
- 1 tbsp honey
- 2 tbsp lemon juice
- ½ cup blueberry

Instructions:

1. Add all ingredients to in a mason jar, and stir them.
2. Mix, cover, and put in the fridge overnight.
3. Eat it chilled in the morning. Add additional yoghurt or blueberries on top of the oats before serving.

Why it's kidney-safe:

The food contains well-balanced calcium, fibre and potassium. The lemon adds citric acid, a stone inhibitor.

2. Savoury Veggie Scramble

Ingredients:

- 2 eggs or egg whites
- ½ cup chopped capsicum
- ¼ cup diced zucchini
- 1 tbsp chopped parsley or basil
- Pinch of turmeric and black pepper

Instructions:

1. Roast the vegetables in a non-stick pan with no stick.
2. Add the eggs and mix till they are cooked.
3. Add herbs on top and serve on whole-grain toast.

Why it's kidney-safe:

High in potassium and magnesium; low in oxalate and sodium.

Lunches

3. Lentil and Cucumber Salad

Ingredients:

- 1 cup cooked lentils (rinsed if canned)
- ½ cucumber, diced
- 1 small carrot, grated
- 1 tbsp olive oil
- Juice of ½ lemon
- Pinch of cumin and salt
- Fresh mint or parsley (optional)

Instructions:

1. Put all the ingredients in a bowl.
2. Toss and serve.

Why it's kidney-safe:

It includes plant protein, potassium, fibre, and citrus.

4. Vegetarian Hummus Wrap

Ingredients:

- 1 whole grain wrap
- 2 tbsp hummus
- ¼ avocado, sliced
- Leaves of romaine lettuce or arugula
- 2 tablespoons of grated cheese or tofu
- Tomato slices

Instructions:

1. Spread hummus in an even manner on the wrap.
2. Place the rest of the ingredients in place and roll tightly.

Why it's kidney-safe:

Leafy greens with low oxalate, moderate salt, and a good calcium balance.

Dinners

5. Lemon-Garlic Baked Salmon

Ingredients:

- 2 salmon fillets (120–150g each)
- Juice of 1 lemon
- 2 cloves garlic, minced
- 1 tbsp olive oil
- Fresh dill or parsley

Instructions:

1. Set the oven to 180°C (350°F).
2. Put the fish in a baking dish or foil. Add lemon, garlic, oil, and herbs on top.
3. Bake for 15 to 18 minutes, or until flaky.

Why it's kidney-safe:

Omega-3s assist with the maintenance of anti-inflammatory response. The citric acid in the lemons are a stone inhibitor.

6. Veggie Stir-Fry with Tofu

Ingredients:

- 1 cup broccoli florets
- 1 cup sliced carrots
- ½ red capsicum, sliced
- ½ block firm tofu (calcium-set), cubed
- 1 tbsp low-sodium soy sauce
- 1 teaspoon of sesame oil
- Fresh ginger grate

Instructions:

1. Stir fry the tofu until it turns golden then add the remaining vegetables
2. Season with the soy sauce and stir

Serve with: Ideal serving with brown rice and quinoa.

Why it's kidney-safe:

Tofu is rich with calcium while vegetables provide a fibre source.

Snacks & Sips

7. Kidney-Friendly Smoothie

Ingredients:

- Half banana
- One tablespoon of honey
- One tablespoon of crushed flaxseed

- One cup of oat milk or cow's milk
- Half lime juice
- A tiny handful of blueberries

Instructions:

1. Put ingredients in a blender.
2. Chill before serving.

Why it's safe for the kidneys:

This smoothie combines fruits that are naturally low in oxalates and are high in citrate, fibre and healthy fats.

8. Citrus Water for Daily Sipping

Ingredients:

- 1 litre water
- Juice of ½ lemon
- Pieces of cucumber or fresh mint

Instructions:

1. Mix in a bottle.
2. Keep it cool and drink it all day.

Why it's kidney-safe:

Raises citrate levels and increases hydration to flush out any stone promoting proteins!

Recipe Tips for Long-Term Success

- **Focus on real food**, not restriction
- **Batch cook staples** like lentils, brown rice, or roasted veggies to save time.
- **Keep lemon juice or citrus wedges** on hand to add to water.
- **Read labels**: Check sodium content on pre-packaged items.

In the following chapter, we'll look at things outside of the kitchen that affect stone risk, such as sleep, exercise, and stress. These things are equally as important as nutrition.

Chapter 6:
Lifestyle Modification

What you eat isn't the only thing that might cause kidney stones. Your lifestyle can also play a role. Your stone risk can all be affected by stress, sleep, exercise, and even your daily schedule.

This chapter will talk about the practices that might help you avoid getting stones in the future and how to make them a part of your life.

1. Regular exercise

Regular exercise helps you keep your weight healthy, lowers your blood pressure, and helps your body use insulin more efficiently. These benefits lower the risk of developing some types of kidney stones, such as uric acid stones and calcium oxalate stones.

Aim for:

- **150 minutes per week** of moderate activity (like brisk walking or cycling)
- **Strength training** 2 times per week for muscle development

Why it works:

- Physical activity **lowers urinary calcium excretion**
- Exercise improves hydration awareness and reduces obesity—a key risk factor
- Sweating (with rehydration!) flushes out toxins gently

Pro tip: If you sweat a lot, drink right after working out to keep hydrated.

2. Maintain a Healthy Weight

Being overweight or obese will increase your chances of getting stones due to the following reasons:

- Increased **uric acid production**
- **Insulin resistance**, which affects how the kidneys process calcium and oxalate
- Chronic inflammation, which affects your urinary pH

It can also help even if you lose 5 to 10 per cent of your body weight in case you are overweight. **But avoid crash diets**—rapid weight loss, especially high-protein or keto-style, can *increase* stone risk.

3. Manage Stress Levels

Stress doesn't directly cause kidney stones—but it influences:

- **Hormonal balance** (like cortisol), which affects kidney function
- **Sleep quality**, which impacts metabolism and inflammation
- **Emotional eating** or dehydration (people often drink less water under stress)

Ways to reduce stress:

- Mindful breathing or meditation (5–10 minutes daily)
- Daily walks in nature
- Short digital detox periods (away from screens)
- Journaling or gratitude practice

Even small stress-reduction habits can shift your nervous system into a kidney-friendly, anti-inflammatory state.

4. Sleep for Stone Prevention

Poor sleep increases stone risk via:

- Hormonal disruption (especially cortisol and insulin)
- Increased inflammation and blood pressure
- Reduced motivation to hydrate or eat well

Aim for:

- **7–9 hours** of quality sleep per night
- Consistent sleep/wake times

- A calming pre-bed routine (e.g., dim lights, no screens 1 hour before bed)

5. Stay Hydrated—All Day, Every Day

Hydration is more than chugging water all at once. The **timing and consistency** of your fluid intake matter.

Tips to hydrate smartly:

- Start with **2 cups of water first thing in the morning**
- Sip throughout the day—don't wait for thirst
- Keep a **water bottle** with you at all times
- Flavour water naturally with **citrus, cucumber, or mint**
- Track your **urine colour**—aim for pale yellow to clear

Target: 2.5–3 litres of fluid per day, unless otherwise directed by your doctor. (More if exercising or in hot climates.)

6. Watch for Medication Side Effects

Some common medications can increase stone risk:

- **Calcium or vitamin D supplements** in excess can raise calcium levels
- **Antacids with calcium** or high doses of vitamin C

Always review medications with your doctor—especially if you've had a stone before.

7. Avoid Extreme Fads

Crash diets, juice cleanses, high-protein regimens, or "detoxes" can unbalance your chemistry and **trigger stones** by:

- Dropping citrate levels
- Spiking oxalate intake
- Overloading your body with protein or supplements

The best "detox" is:

- Consistent water intake
- High-fibre, low-sodium eating
- Plenty of plant-based meals
- Balanced movement and rest

Lifestyle Summary Checklist

Habit	Kidney-Friendly Action
Hydration	2.5–3L daily, evenly spread
Sleep	7–9 hours/night, consistent schedule
Activity	150+ mins/week movement
Stress	Daily 5–10 min relaxation
Weight	Aim for a BMI in the healthy range (20-25)
Avoid	Crash diets, excess supplements
Monitor	Medication effects with your doctor

Chapter 7:
The 4 Week Stone Free Plan

This plan provides general guidance only and should be adapted with your doctor if you have medical conditions or concerns.

Now you know the concepts, it is time to put it all in action. The following plan aims to change your habits to prevent kidney stones over 4 weeks. It aims to be sustainable!

How the Plan Works

- **Week 1: Increasing Hydration**
- **Week 2: Nutrition Reset**
- **Week 3: Lifestyle Sync**
- **Week 4: Long-Term Momentum**

Week 1: Hydration & Foundations

Goals:

1. Consume at least 2.5 to 3 litres of water per day
2. Identify and reduce **1 high-risk food habit**

Daily Checklist:

- Drank 2.5–3L of fluid
- Had lemon or citrus water
- Urine was light yellow
- Avoided soda or high-oxalate food
- Ate 1 serving of low-oxalate veggies

Tips:

- Set alarms or use a hydration app
- Track your urine colour—it's your best hydration gauge

Week 2: Nutrition Reset

Goals:

1. Eat **3 calcium-rich foods daily**
2. Include **low-oxalate fruits and veggies** at each meal
3. Make **2 healthy food swaps** (see Chapter 4)

Daily Checklist:

- Ate 3+ calcium-containing foods
- Paired calcium with oxalate-rich foods (if eaten)

- Included lemon or lime
- Avoided processed snacks or salt-heavy meals

Week 3: Lifestyle Sync

Goals:

1. Exercise for at least **30 minutes/day**
2. Get **7-9 hours of sleep** nightly
3. Add a **5-minute daily de-stress ritual**

Daily Checklist:

- Got 30+ mins movement
- Slept 7-9 hours
- Practised stress relief (deep breathing, walking, meditation)
- Ate at regular times
- Stayed hydrated throughout the day

Tips:

- Turn off screens 1 hour before bed
- Use a sleep or fitness tracker if helpful

Week 4: Long-Term Momentum

Goals:

1. Review your food & water patterns
2. Identify **3 habits to keep** and **1 to improve**
3. Plan a **kidney-friendly week** on your own

Daily Checklist:

- Continue regular fluid intake
- Ate 3+ kidney safe meals
- Improved sleep and exercise pattern
- Reflected on your progress

Tips:

- Use a journal or app to track your meals and fluid intake
- Build a rotating meal plan with 3 breakfasts, 3 lunches, 3 dinners
- Ask yourself weekly: *What's working? What needs support?*

Final Thoughts for Your 4 Week Plan

- Small, consistent habits **lower your stone forming risk dramatically**
- Most people see results in **energy, digestion, and hydration** within 2 weeks
- Revisit the chapters anytime you feel off track—this is a toolkit to empower you!

Chapter 8:
Staying Stonefree for Life

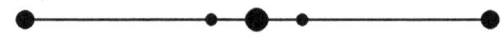

You have come to the end of the book – congratulations for the taking the first step! Prevention is not a one-time exercise but a series of small habits to take care of your kidney health. You have learnt the following:

1. Stay Hydrated—Always

Water is your biggest weapon. Keep it simple:

- **Track trends, not perfection:** Aim for 2.5–3 litres most days. A few off-days won't undo your progress.
- **Watch for triggers:** Travel, exercise, or illness can reduce your intake—plan extra fluids during these times.

2. Revisit the 4 Week Plan

Think of the 4 Week Plan as your **reset button**. If you slip into old habits (as everyone does), go back to:

- **Week 1** for hydration
- **Week 2** to review your food choices
- **Week 3-4** to reinforce lifestyle stability

Repeat the full plan every 6-12 months or **after a stone episode**, if needed.

3. Check in with your General Practitioner or Urologist and know when to be concerned

You can have setbacks without realising it, even when you have done a good job. Frequent check-ins with your general practitioner or urologist can be useful. Seek a medical opinion if you experience the following:

- Flank or lower back pain
- Blood in urine
- Pain with urination or cloudy urine
- Fever or chills with urinary symptoms

4. Celebrate the Wins

Improving your kidney health also means improving your OVERALL HEALTH! Not only have you reduced the risk of getting kidney stones, you have also built good habits to improve your lifestyle, mood and general wellbeing!

A Stone-Free Life Is Possible

Kidney stones are frustrating and painful however they are also **preventable**.

By following the principles in this book - hydration, food balance, exercise, and habit change - you have already taken powerful action to improve your kidney health.

You do not need to be perfect – you just need to be aware, have small positive habits and be kind to your body.

Here's to a life free of pain, full of energy, and guided by choices that work with your body—not against it.

About the Author

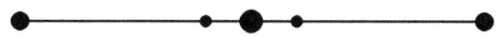

Dr Anthony Dat is an Australian Urologist with extensive experience in urinary stone disease. He completed surgical training and obtained Fellowship of the Royal Australasian College of Surgeons (FRACS) in 2022. He subsequently completed further advanced fellowship training in Uro-Oncology and Robotic Surgery at Oxford University NHS Trust, United Kingdom. He has extensive experience in all facets of urinary stone surgery and management. In addition to his clinical expertise, he is passionate about health promotion and population health. Through his writing, Dr Dat aims to bridge the gap between specialist knowledge and everyday practice—providing clear, actionable strategies that help readers reduce their stone risk and make long-term changes for better kidney health.

Further information can be obtained from his website
www.daturology.com.au.

Any further queries can be directed to
admin@daturology.com.au.

www.ingramcontent.com/pod-product-compliance
Lightning Source LLC
Chambersburg PA
CBHW060033040426
42333CB00042B/2436